THE *Skinny*
BREAD MACHINE
RECIPE BOOK

You may also enjoy The Skinny Soup Maker Recipe Book. The perfect companion to The Skinny Bread Machine Recipe Book.

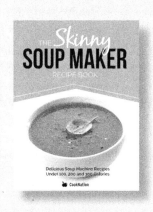

The Skinny Bread Machine Recipe Book
70 Simple, Lower Calorie, Healthy Breads... Baked To Perfection In Your Bread Maker

A Bell & Mackenzie Publishing Limited Publication.
First published in 2013 by Bell & Mackenzie Publishing Limited.

ISBN 978-1-909855-20-5

A CIP catalogue record of this book is available from the British Library

Disclaimer
The information and advice in this book is intended as a guide only. If using the recipes as part of a diet, any individual should independently seek the advice of a doctor or health professional before embarking on any diet or weight loss plan. We do not recommend a calorie controlled diet if you are pregnant, breastfeeding, elderly or under 18 years of age. Some recipes may contain nuts or traces of nuts. Those suffering from any allergies associated with nuts should avoid any recipes containing nuts or nut based oils.avoid any recipes containing nuts or nut based oils.

Contents

Introduction   7
Bread Science   9
Which Bread Machine   11
Bread Machine Cycles   13
Tips   15
Bread Improver   18
Flour   19
Troubleshooting   19
Basic Breads   **23**
Standard White Loaf   24
Standard Wholemeal Loaf   25
White Breads   **27**
Cumin Bread   28
Honey Fig Loaf   29
'Chocolate' Chilli Bread   30
Horseradish & Mustard Bread   31
Tarragon & Mozzarella Cheese   32
Red Pesto Bread   33
Cranberry Bread   34
Cheese & Pepper Bread   35
Italian Semolina Bread   36
Wheatgerm White   37
Double Dairy Bread   38
Light Milk Loaf   39
Spiced Butternut Squash Bread   40
Pink Beetroot Bread   41
Polenta Bread   42
Honey & Pumpkin Seed Bread   43
Mozzarella & Basil Bread   44
Italian Bread   45
Fat Free Yoghurt & Chilli Bread   46
Garlic & Oregano Bread   47

Contents

Sundried Tomato Bread   48
Four Herb Bread   49
Mediterranean Rosemary Bread   50
Olive Bread   51
Thyme & Lemon Bread   52
Red Onion Bread   53
Indian Spiced Bread   54
Chorizo & Mozzarella Bread   55
Double Seed Lemon Bread   56
Bacon & Mustard Bread   57
Wholemeal & Brown Breads   **59**
Granary Grain Bread   60
Raisin & Pecan Bread   61
Caraway Rye Bread   62
Granola Loaf   63
Sweet Fennel Bread   64
Orange & Poppy Seed Bread   65
Rye & Cocoa Bread   66
Honey & Pumpkin Seed Loaf   67
Cinnamon & Carrot Bread   68
Almond & Syrup Bread   69
Oaty Bread   70
Barley Milk Bread   71
Triple Seed Bread   72
Granary & Stout Loaf   73
Lemon & Parsley Bread   74
Walnut Bread   75
Granary Linseed Bread   76
German Seed Bread   77
Dried Chilli Bread   78
Malthouse Bread   79
Barleycorn Flour Loaf   80

Contents

Russian Bread	82
Buckwheat Loaf	82
Sweet Breads	**83**
Banana Bread	84
Festive Apple Bread	85
Pineapple & Coconut Bread	86
Dried Cherry Loaf	87
Mixed Fruit & Double Spice Loaf	88
Macadamia & Syrup Loaf	89
Raisin Gingerbread	90
Apricot & Cinnamon Bread	91
Peanut Butter Bread	92
Honey Porridge Loaf	93
Gluten Free Breads	**95**
Rice Bread	96
Cinnamon Mixed Fruit Loaf	97
Mixed Seed Bread	98
Besan Bread	99
Other CookNation Titles	**103**

Introduction

Bread – one of the world's oldest foods and a staple part of our diet. A food which compliments a myriad of dishes but just as comforting and 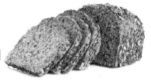 delicious all on its own. The aroma of freshly baked bread is like no other and it fills your home with warmth and goodness. We all love bread, yet increasingly many are feeling that it is becoming difficult to eat as part of a healthy diet.

Bread has had some bad press mostly due to its high levels of carbohydrates. Our bodies convert carbohydrates present in wheat flour to sugar, quickly producing sugar spikes. Blood sugar levels increase, which means after a few hours the body craves more carbs and you may find yourself searching for another quick sugar-rush to satisfy your craving.

In addition many store bought loaves, particularly white breads, are low in nutrients. The refining process of the flour, which involves bleaching, strips all the essential vitamins and minerals leaving little in the way of goodness. This, coupled with the popularity of low carb diets and gluten/digestive issues, have added to the negative press for our much-loved loaf.

So, can you really eat bread as part of a healthy diet? Yes of course you can.

Bread can be a great source of fibre, vitamin B, healthy fats and, while high carbohydrates can be a problem, they do provide energy which fuels our bodies on a daily basis. While bread may never be at the top of anyone's diet list as the healthiest, most nutritious food in the world, it can, with a little care, attention, common sense and adjustment, still be a healthier part of your diet - compared to many store bought loaves.

For each of our skinny bread machine recipes, we have taken the traditional ingredients and, where possible, replaced them with alternatives which are either lower in calories, sugar, salt or saturated fats. It is important to remember however that the baking of bread is a science and therefore replacing ingredients can and will directly affect the performance of your finished loaf. Often many ingredients such as a teaspoon of sugar and salt are entirely necessary for the bread to bake so there is only so far a 'skinny' loaf can go!

To keep things as skinny as possible we have opted to replace some of the more traditional bread ingredients such as full fat butter, milk and cheese with some of the following more health conscious options:

• Low fat olive spread	• Olive oil
• 'Half spoon' Silver Spoon sugar	• Unsweetened cocoa powder
• Honey	• Sunflower oil
• Agave nectar	• Vegetable oil
• Reduced fat cheeses	• Low fat peanut butter
• Fat free Greek yoghurt	• Lean trimmed bacon
• Skimmed milk	

Each of the recipes have been tried and tested to make perfect homemade bread in your bread machine. The freshly baked bread you make will look and taste great and you'll be happy you've done your best to bake a healthier loaf for you and your family.

Bread Science

It is often said that "cooking is an art whilst baking is a science" - and not a truer word was said. Baking requires a chemical reaction, which changes the components whilst being baked. The exact measurements and ratios must be correct to get the best outcome...in other words it's an exact science.

The good news is you needn't be an artist or a scientist to make a great loaf of bread in your bread machine. It is however helpful to understand the basis of the bio-chemical process which magically makes bread.

One of the key ingredients of most bread making is yeast. Yeast is a type of fungus made up of single cells, which reproduce and can convert sugar into alcohol and carbon dioxide. Carbon dioxide is what gives bread its light, airy texture while the alcohol, when cooked and burned off, gives bread its distinctive flavour.

Yeast when added to flour and water causes a chemical reaction. Starch that is present in flour is turned into a type of sugar called maltose. This process is what makes the bread rise by producing carbon dioxide. The addition of more sugar to a recipe will help this process further, but too much will spoil it.

Yeast is an organism, which becomes more active in warmer temperatures. This why in a traditional hand-prepared loaf, the bread dough is placed in a warm oven to react faster.

Wheat flour, when mixed with water, forms the dough which becomes elastic in its texture when kneaded. This is because the kneading process of the flour and water releases a protein known as gluten. Gluten allows the bread to capture the carbon dioxide produced by the yeast giving a light, spongy loaf (look at the air bubbles you can see when breaking a fresh loaf of bread).

This is why it is so important to be accurate with your measurements. Each recipe lists the correct ratio of ingredients in relation to each other to make the chemical reaction (science) just right.

Similarly, the sequence of adding ingredients to your bread machine is equally important. For example, yeast when in contact with water will begin activating too early and can become ineffective if it comes into direct contact with salt and sugar before the mixing cycle begins. This is why we list the ingredients in specific order i.e. starting with water and generally ending with yeast. Altering the sequence of ingredients will affect how your loaf turns out.

Luckily for us the bread machine makes the amazing chemical process very easy. All we have to do is adhere carefully to the measurements, set the cycle and wait for the machine to make a perfect homemade loaf.

Which Bread Machine?

You may already own a bread machine, are perhaps thinking about replacing an older appliance or are contemplating purchasing for the first time. There are many different manufacturers and models on the market but all work using the same principles.

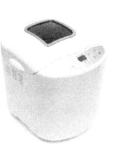

Cost

Prices range from as little as £45.00 up to £300.00 or $65.00 up to $500.00. Consider your budget.

Features

Think about the features of a bread machine that you are likely to use most often. Many new models offer specific cycles for jam making, cake baking & gluten free/yeast free bread (these cycles are generally shorter because less time is needed for mixing and rising due to the absence of gluten and yeast). If you are unlikely to use these settings then a more straightforward traditional bread machine may be better suited to your needs. To follow are the most common features included in modern bread machines.

Size matters

What size of loaf will you be making? The majority of machines will offer the capability to bake 450g, 750g and 1kg loaves (1lb, 1.5lb & 2.2lb). Smaller machines may only make 450g loaves.

The majority of recipes in The Skinny Bread Machine Recipe Book are for 750g (1.5lb) sized loaves.

Timer Delay

This enables you to add the ingredients to your bread machine and set the timer to start baking. So, if you like to wake up to the wonderful aroma of freshly baked bread, you can prepare the night before. However it is important not to use fresh ingredients such as milk, eggs & cheese, which may perish at room temperature.

Fruit & Nut Dispenser

Standard on most machines, this handy addition will automatically add ingredients at the right point during a cycle. It is just as easy to add these ingredients by hand at the required time (if your machine doesn't have a dispenser it should have an alarm/prompt to let you know when to add the extra ingredients manually). All our recipes assume that your bread machine has a dispenser or an audible prompt to let you know when to add the additional ingredients.

Digital Display

Most machines will have these are standard but it's always worth checking as it will allow you to see at a glance which stage of the baking process your loaf is going through, which cycle you have selected, crust colour and how much time remains of the baking process.

Inspection Window

Most people like to observe their bread as it goes through the magical process of mixing, rising and baking. If you are one of these people then make sure you choose a model with an inspection window.

Power Interruption

Some machines include a facility to compensate for a short power cut to the cycle. The cycle will pick up from the last point when power resumes and carry on the process. If the power has been off for longer the 20 minutes we would recommend discarding contents and starting again.

Crust Colour

As standard most appliances will offer either light, medium or dark crust options.

Reserach Your Appliance

As with any new purchase we recommend you thoroughly research the products before buying. Search for recommendations and pay particular attention to all customer reviews...good and bad! This will help you make an informed decision on your bread machine. Be sure to investigate the manufacturers guarantees and after sales service too.

Bread Machine Cycles

To follow are the most common cycles offered with bread machines. Many come as standard but you should consider which of these you are most likely to use when selecting your appliance.

Basic

Primarily used for basic white breads with less rising cycles and shorter baking time.

Turbo/Rapid Cycle

If you need your bread in a hurry then this cycle usually

completes in around 90 minutes. The rising time is reduced which will produce a denser loaf. Generally this cycle is less suitable for wholemeal breads.

Gluten & Yeast Free Cycle
Again a shorter cycle where less rising time is needed due to the absence of gluten/yeast.

Wheat Cycle
When making bread using predominantly whole wheat, rye, oats or bran, the wheat cycle allows the flour and grains to absorb liquid for a longer period making them softer and able to combine more easily. It also increases the rising time to allow for the heavier ingredients.

French Bread Cycle
For loaves with a thicker, crunchier crust.

Sweet Bread Cycle
The cycle is increased to allow for additional kneading and rising and the temperature is set lower than that of a traditional loaf to prevent additional ingredients, particularly sugar based, from burning.

Dough Cycle
If you wish to shape your dough, for example into round bread rolls, this cycle will mix, knead and allow the dough to rise. You can them remove the dough, cut, shape and bake in a conventional oven.

Bake only
If you plan to make fruitcakes or gingerbread this is a great

feature to have.

Other Cycles
Jam – mixes and heats ingredients for jams
Cakes (many manufactures recommend pre-packaged cake mixes)
Pasta Dough
Pizza Dough

Tips
• Check your bread as it kneads. Most bread machines have an inspection window so you can watch progress. Don't be afraid to pause the cycle during the mixing and kneading stage by lifting the lid if need be. Sometimes dough or flour can stick to the sides of 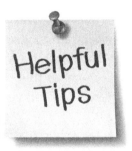 the loaf tin. If this happens simply use a plastic spatula to scrape from the sides of the bread pan then close the lid and resume the cycle. This will not affect the end result of your bread. You should not lift the lid during the rising/proofing or baking stages.

• You may need to add a little more water to your dough if you feel it looks to dry. Add only a tablespoon at a time. Conversely if the dough looks too wet you may need to add a little more flour.

• When using a delayed cycle do not use fresh ingredients such as eggs, milk, cheese etc. Leaving these ingredients at room temperature for several hours before baking can cause bacteria to grow and therefore pose a risk of food poisoning.

• Add the bread ingredients exactly in the order stated in each recipe. This is important and altering can affect how your loaf turns out. Yeast, when in contact with water, will activate too early and also can become ineffective if it comes into direct contact with salt and sugar.

• Whenever possible, remove your freshly baked loaf from the bread pan as soon as the cycle has finished and allow to cool on a wire rack. The moisture in the loaf needs to evaporate to give you a firm loaf. Leaving the bread in the bread machine will trap moisture and make your loaf soggy. Remember that the loaf tin will be very hot so wear oven gloves to remove.

• If you find the base of your loaf feels a little too soft when removed from the bread pan, you can pop it upside down in a preheated oven (175ºC/350ºF) for 10 mins to firm it up.

• Using accurate measurements is really important. Bread making is a science. Avoid rounding off teaspoons or tablespoons as this will alter the end result. Use a kitchen measuring spoon for accuracy. You will be surprised at the difference between a teaspoon and a measuring spoon and this could make or break the quality of your loaf. For flour, use accurate kitchen scales.

• Measure water using electronic scales if you have them. This is much more accurate than a traditional measuring jug. 1 ml of water weighs 1 gram.

• Always use tepid water when adding ingredients, not cold or hot. Optimum temperature should be between 20-25 ºC/68-77ºF.

• If your tap water has high chlorine content, use filtered water instead. Chlorine can affect the performance of yeast.

• When adding low fat spread, cut into small cubes so that it blends well with the ingredients.

• If you find your loaf sinks, it may be because the dough was too wet. Try using less liquid next time.

• Remove the loaf tin from the machine before adding the ingredients. This will prevent any spillages onto the baking element.

• Remove any spillages from your loaf tin before switching on your bread machine. Clean off any spillages on the cooking element with a damp cloth. Make sure your machine is turned off and that the element is completely cool before doing this.

• Regularly wipe down and clean your fruit/nut dispenser. It's easy to forget about this area.

• Allow your loaf to completely cool before slicing. This will make slicing much easier. Slicing while still warm can allow too much moisture into the loaf.

• Place your loaf on its side and cut using a bread knife in a sawing motion. Cut thin slices. Thick doorstep sized wedges will obviously increase your calorie intake.

• If your loaf does not easily come out of the bread pan after baking, use a plastic spatula around the edges of the loaf to help release it. Do not use metal utensils as this will damage the non-stick surface of your bread pan.

• Make sure all ingredients are fresh. Store all ingredients, including flour, in air-tight containers and regularly check use-by dates.

• If using individual portions of packet fast action yeast, discard any left over yeast. Yeast will begin to degenerate once opened and will become ineffective if you use it for your next loaf.

• If freezing, allow to cool completely, slice, then wrap in a plastic freezer bag.

• Always read the manufacturers instructions before using your machine for the first time.

Bread Improver

Bread improver comes in a powdered form and is used to improve the quality of the crumb, texture, crust and volume of your loaf. Many manufactures of bread machines recommend its use when baking bread.

There is much discussion as to whether or not it is needed, or indeed makes a valuable improvement to the finished loaf. It is not an essential ingredient and for the purpose of baking healthier loaves we do not include bread improver in any of our recipes.

Flour

Good quality flour will make a difference to the quality of your bread. Strong bread flours will achieve the best results in your bread machine. The majority of our recipes use either strong white bread flour, strong wholemeal flour or a combination of both.

Wholemeal flour retains more nutrients than white flour. Brown loaves tend to be heavier and have a stronger flavour than their white counterparts. Your brown loaf may feel denser, this is normal.

Adding nuts and seeds to a wholewheat loaf can increase flavour and provide a good source of extra protein and healthy fats, however they can also be high in calories so if you are watching your weight, bear this in mind.

Troubleshooting

To follow is a list of the most common problems and solutions when baking bread using a bread machine.

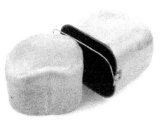

Problem:
• The dough does not rise,
Possible Cause:
• The liquid added was too hot or too cold. It should be tepid between 20-25 ºC/68-77ºF.
• Not enough yeast was added. Make sure your

measurements are accurate.
- Yeast was not fresh and therefore inactive.
- Yeast came into contact with salt prior to mixing.
- Too much salt was added counteracting performance of yeast. Make sure your measurements are accurate.

Problem:
- Bread has risen and fallen over the side of the loaf tin.
Possible Cause:
- Too much dough. Check you have selected the right quantity of ingredients for your loaf and bread machine.
- Too much yeast has caused the bread to over-rise. Make sure your measurements are accurate.
- Not enough sugar. Make sure your measurements are accurate.
- Not enough salt. Salt affects the performance of yeast, too little or too much will have an adverse effect on your loaf.

Problem:
- Bread has collapsed.
Possible Cause:
- Too much yeast has caused the bread to over-rise. Make sure your measurements are accurate.

Problem:
- Bread is heavy.
Possible Cause:
- Not enough liquid.
- Too much flour.
- Flour or yeast is not fresh.
- Make sure ingredients are fresh and quantities are

accurate.

Problem:

• Bread is very dry.

Possible Cause:

• Not enough liquid. Make sure your measurements are accurate.

• If your loaf contains oats, bran, rye or wholegrains it may be that they have soaked up additional liquid. Experiment by adding slightly more liquid or reduce the quantity of grains.

Problem:

• Bread is undercooked in the middle.

Possible Cause:

• Not enough flour.

• Too much liquid.

• Flour is of a poor quality or is not fresh.

Problem:

• Bread crust is burnt.

Possible Cause:

• Too much sugar. Reduce quantity of sugar or sugar-based ingredients. You may also consider using the sweet bread cycle if your machine has one, which will bake your bread at a lower temperature and therefore avoid burning the crust.

• Dark crust has been selected. Select a lighter crust setting.

Problem:

• Crust is not crispy.

Possible Cause:

• Loaf requires a French bread cycle if your machine has one.

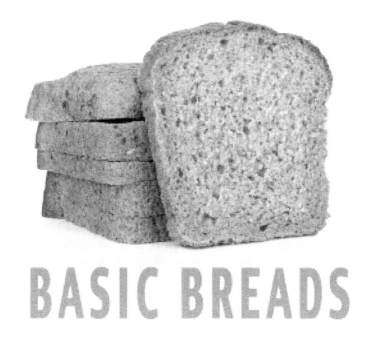

BASIC BREADS

Standard White Loaf
750g Loaf

Ingredients:

315ml water
25g low fat olive spread
1 ½ tsp salt
1 ½ tsp 'half spoon'
Silver Spoon sugar
1 tbsp skimmed milk
powder
600g strong white bread
flour
1 ½ tsp fast action dried
yeast

Method:

• Evenly add all the ingredients to the bread maker.
• Add each ingredient one at a time in the order listed.
• Select the basic program on the bread machine for a 750g loaf.
• Select the crust colour and press start.
• When the baking cycle has finished lift the bread pan out of the machine with oven gloves.
• Turn the baked bread out onto a wire rack to cool.

This is the classic white loaf. Simple & delicious.

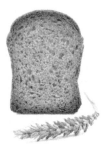

Standard Wholemeal Loaf
750g Loaf

Method:

- Evenly add all the ingredients to the bread maker.
- Add each ingredient one at a time in the order listed.
- Select the basic wheat program on the bread machine for a 750g loaf.
- Select the crust colour and press start.
- When the baking cycle has finished lift the bread pan out of the machine with oven gloves.
- Turn the baked bread out onto a wire rack to cool.

Wholemeal breads are less likely to rise with a rounded top so don't worry is your brown loaves look a little flat compared to the white bread you make.

Ingredients:

320ml water
25g low fat olive spread
1 ½ tsp salt
2 ½ tsp 'half spoon'
Silver Spoon sugar
2 tbsp skimmed milk
powder
540g strong wholemeal
bread flour
1 ½ tsp fast action dried
yeast

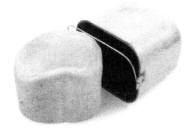

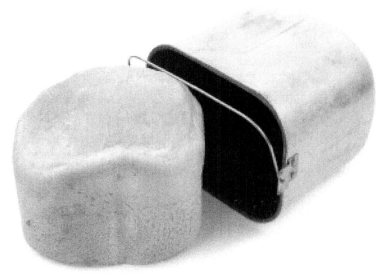

WHITE BREADS

Cumin Bread
750g Loaf

Ingredients:

315ml water
20g low fat olive spread
2 tsp cumin seeds
1 tsp ground cumin
1 ½ tsp salt
1 ½ tsp 'half spoon'
Silver Spoon sugar
1 tbsp skimmed milk
powder
600g strong white bread
flour
1 ½ tsp fast action dried
yeast

Method:

• Evenly add all the ingredients to the bread maker.
• Add each ingredient one at a time in the order listed.
• Select the basic program on the bread machine for a 750g loaf.
• Select the crust colour and press start.
• When the baking cycle has finished lift the bread pan out of the machine with oven gloves.
• Turn the baked bread out onto a wire rack to cool.

Cumin has an unmistakable rich aroma which will fill your kitchen with a lovely warming atmosphere.

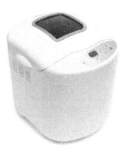

28

Honey Fig Loaf
750g Loaf

Method:

- Evenly add each bread pan ingredient to the bread maker.
- Add one at a time in the order listed.
- Add the chopped figs to the dispenser.
- Select the basic program on the bread machine for a 750g loaf.
- Select the crust colour and press start.
- When the baking cycle has finished lift the bread pan out of the machine with oven gloves.
- Turn the baked bread out onto a wire rack to cool.

Honey is a great natural sweetener which blends really well with the dried figs

Bread Pan Ingredients:

315ml water
20g low fat olive spread
1 ½ tsp runny honey
1 ½ tsp salt
1 tbsp skimmed milk powder
600g strong white bread flour
1 ½ tsp fast action dried yeast

Extra Ingredients:

80g dried chopped figs

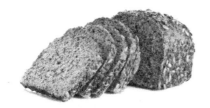

'Chocolate' Chilli Bread
750g Loaf

Ingredients:

315ml water
20g low fat olive spread
1 ½ tsp 'half spoon'
Silver Spoon sugar
1 ½ tsp salt
1 tbsp skimmed milk
powder
1 tbsp unsweetened
cocoa powder
2 tsp chilli powder
600g strong white bread
flour
1 ½ tsp fast action dried
yeast

Method:

• Evenly add all the ingredients to the bread maker.
• Add each ingredient one at a time in the order listed.
• Select the basic program on the bread machine for a 750g loaf.
• Select the crust colour and press start.
• When the baking cycle has finished lift the bread pan out of the machine with oven gloves.
• Turn the baked bread out onto a wire rack to cool.

Cocoa powder is rich in healthy flavonoids, which studies suggest may help protect against coronary heart disease and strokes.

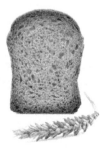

Horseradish & Mustard Bread
750g Loaf

Method:

• Evenly add all the ingredients to the bread maker.
• Add each ingredient one at a time in the order listed.
• Select the basic program on the bread machine for a 750g loaf.
• Select the crust colour and press start.
• When the baking cycle has finished lift the bread pan out of the machine with oven gloves.
• Turn the baked bread out onto a wire rack to cool.

Add a little more mustard powder if you want to give the bread a stronger 'kick'.

Ingredients:

315ml water
20g low fat olive spread
1 ½ tsp salt
1 tbsp horseradish sauce
1 tsp mustard powder
1 ½ tsp 'half spoon' Silver Spoon sugar
1 tbsp skimmed milk powder
600g strong white bread flour
1 ½ tsp fast action dried yeast

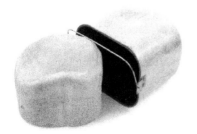

31

Tarragon & Mozzarella Cheese
750g Loaf

Ingredients:

250ml water
150g reduced fat grated mozzarella cheese
1 tbsp dried tarragon
1 ½ tsp 'half spoon' Silver Spoon sugar
1 ½ tsp salt
1 tbsp olive oil
200g strong wholemeal bread flour
250g strong white bread flour
1 ½ tsp fast action dried yeast

Method:

• Evenly add all the ingredients to the bread maker.
• Add each ingredient one at a time in the order listed.
• Select the basic program on the bread machine for a 750g loaf.
• Select the crust colour and press start.
• When the baking cycle has finished lift the bread pan out of the machine with oven gloves.
• Turn the baked bread out onto a wire rack to cool.

All breads need 'fats' to bake properly and olive oil is a great natural option.

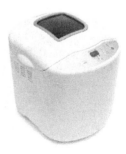

32

Red Pesto Bread
750g Loaf

Method:

• Evenly add each bread pan ingredient to the bread maker.
• Add one at a time in the order listed.
• Add the chopped olives to the dispenser.
• Select the basic program on the bread machine for a 750g loaf.
• Select the crust colour and press start.
• When the baking cycle has finished lift the bread pan out of the machine with oven gloves.
• Turn the baked bread out onto a wire rack to cool.

The pesto alone should provide enough 'fats' for this loaf without the need for additional oil.

Bread Pan Ingredients:

315ml water
1 tbsp red pesto
1 ½ tsp salt
1 ½ tsp 'half spoon' Silver Spoon sugar
2 tbsp skimmed milk powder
600g strong white bread flour
1 ½ tsp fast action dried yeast

Extra Ingredients:

3 tbsp finely chopped green olives

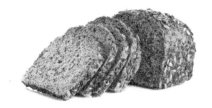

Cranberry Bread
750g Loaf

Bread Pan Ingredients:

315ml water
20g low fat olive spread
40g polenta
1 ½ tsp 'half spoon' Silver Spoon sugar
1 ½ tsp salt
1 tbsp skimmed milk powder
560g strong white bread flour
1 ½ tsp fast action dried yeast

Extra Ingredients:

80g dried chopped cranberries

Method:

• Evenly add each bread pan ingredient to the bread maker.
• Add one at a time in the order listed.
• Add the cranberries to the dispenser.
• Select the basic program on the bread machine for a 750g loaf.
• Select the crust colour and press start.
• When the baking cycle has finished lift the bread pan out of the machine with oven gloves.
• Turn the baked bread out onto a wire rack to cool.

Cranberries are rich in vitamin C, dietary fibre & manganese.

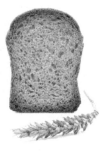

Cheese & Pepper Bread
750g Loaf

Method:

• Evenly add all the ingredients to the bread maker.
• Add each ingredient one at a time in the order listed.
• Select the basic program on the bread machine for a 750g loaf.
• Select the crust colour and press start.
• When the baking cycle has finished lift the bread pan out of the machine with oven gloves.
• Turn the baked bread out onto a wire rack to cool.

Ingredients:

1 tbsp olive oil
1 ½ tsp 'half spoon'
Silver Spoon sugar
250ml water
1 tsp freshly milled
black pepper
75g low fat grated
Cheddar cheese
425g strong white bread
flour
1 ½ tsp fast action dried
yeast

You could substitute the cheddar cheese for any other low fat cheese you prefer.

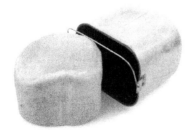

Italian Semolina Bread
750g Loaf

Ingredients:

200ml water
6 tbsp olive oil
1 tsp salt
1 tsp 'half spoon' Silver Spoon sugar
150g semolina
300g strong white bread flour
1 ¼ tsp fast action dried yeast

Method:

• Evenly add all the ingredients to the bread maker.
• Add each ingredient one at a time in the order listed.
• Select the basic program on the bread machine for a 750g loaf.
• Select the crust colour and press start.
• When the baking cycle has finished lift the bread pan out of the machine with oven gloves.
• Turn the baked bread out onto a wire rack to cool.

The semolina makes this a fairly heavy loaf which will not rise hugely, but tastes great!

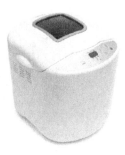

Wheatgerm White
750g Loaf

Method:

- Evenly add all the ingredients to the bread maker.
- Add each ingredient one at a time in the order listed.
- Select the basic program on the bread machine for a 750g loaf.
- Select the crust colour and press start.
- When the baking cycle has finished lift the bread pan out of the machine with oven gloves.
- Turn the baked bread out onto a wire rack to cool.

Agave syrup, also known as agave nectar, is a wonderful natural sweetener.

Ingredients:

275ml water
2 tbsp vegetable oil
1 ½ tsp salt
1 tbsp agave syrup
400g strong white bread flour
60g wheatgerm
2 ½ tsp fast action dried yeast

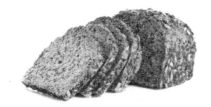

Double Dairy Bread
750g Loaf

Ingredients:

1 free range egg
1 free range egg yolk
25g low fat olive spread
200ml skimmed milk
1 ½ tsp 'half spoon'
Silver Spoon sugar
1 tsp salt
475g strong white bread
flour
1 tsp fast action dried
yeast

Method:

• Evenly add all the ingredients to the bread maker.
• Add each ingredient one at a time in the order listed.
• Select the basic program on the bread machine for a 750g loaf.
• Select the crust colour and press start.
• When the baking cycle has finished lift the bread pan out of the machine with oven gloves.
• Turn the baked bread out onto a wire rack to cool.

Using skimmed milk in this recipe helps reduce the calories.

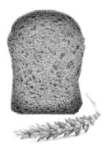

Light Milk Loaf
750g Loaf

Method:

• Evenly add all the ingredients to the bread maker.
• Add each ingredient one at a time in the order listed.
• Select the basic program on the bread machine for a 750g loaf.
• Select the crust colour and press start.
• When the baking cycle has finished lift the bread pan out of the machine with oven gloves.
• Turn the baked bread out onto a wire rack to cool.

Ingredients:

310ml skimmed milk
25g low fat olive spread
1 ½ tsp salt
2 tsp 'half spoon' Silver Spoon sugar
600g strong white bread flour
1 ½ tsp fast action dried yeast

You could use coconut oil instead of olive spread for a slightly different twist.

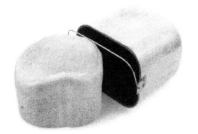

39

Spiced Butternut Squash Bread
750g Loaf

Ingredients:

300ml water
20g low fat olive spread
150g finely chopped butternut squash flesh
1 tsp cinnamon
1 tsp nutmeg
1 ½ tsp salt
1 ½ tsp 'half spoon' Silver Spoon sugar
1 tbsp skimmed milk powder
520g strong white bread flour
1 ½ tsp fast action dried yeast

Method:

• Place the chopped butternut squash in a bowl. Add 1 tbsp spoon of water, cover with clingfilm and microwave for 3 mins. Drain and pat dry.
• Evenly add all the ingredients to the bread maker, one at a time in the order listed.
• Select the basic program on the bread machine for a 750g loaf.
• Select the crust colour and press start.
• When the baking cycle has finished lift the bread pan out of the machine with oven gloves.
• Turn the baked bread out onto a wire rack to cool.

You could use pumpkin rather than butternut squash if you prefer.

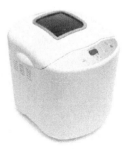

Pink Beetroot Bread
750g Loaf

Method:

- Evenly add all the ingredients to the bread maker.
- Add each ingredient one at a time in the order listed.
- Select the basic program on the bread machine for a 750g loaf.
- Select the crust colour and press start.
- When the baking cycle has finished lift the bread pan out of the machine with oven gloves.
- Turn the baked bread out onto a wire rack to cool.

This bread has a vibrant colour, which will brighten up any kitchen table.

Ingredients:

1 vacuum packed cooked beetroot, finely chopped
1 tbsp beetroot juice (there should be some in the packaging you can scoop out)
1 tbsp dried rosemary
315ml water
20g low fat olive spread
1 ½ tsp salt
1 ½ tsp 'half spoon' Silver Spoon sugar
1 tbsp skimmed milk powder
600g strong white bread flour
1 ½ tsp fast action dried yeast

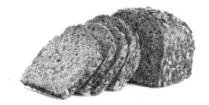

Polenta Bread
750g Loaf

Bread Pan Ingredients:

300ml water
20g low fat olive spread
50g polenta
1 ½ tsp 'half spoon' Silver Spoon sugar
1 ½ tsp salt
1 tbsp skimmed milk powder
560g strong white bread flour
1 ½ tsp fast action dried yeast

Extra Ingredients:

80g tinned sweetcorn, drained
1 tbsp dried oregano

Method:

• Evenly add each bread pan ingredient to the bread maker.
• Add one at a time in the order listed.
• Add the extra ingredients to the dispenser.
• Select the basic program on the bread machine for a 750g loaf.
• Select the crust colour and press start.
• When the baking cycle has finished lift the bread pan out of the machine with oven gloves.
• Turn the baked bread out onto a wire rack to cool.

Derived from maize, polenta is a lovely cornmeal available almost everywhere.

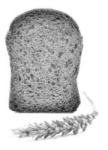

Honey & Pumpkin Seed Bread
750g Loaf

Method:

• Evenly add each bread-pan ingredient to the bread maker.
• Add one at a time in the order listed.
• Add the pumpkin seeds to the dispenser.
• Select the basic program on the bread machine for a 750g loaf.
• Select the crust colour and press start.
• When the baking cycle has finished lift the bread pan out of the machine with oven gloves.
• Turn the baked bread out onto a wire rack to cool.

Use good quality pure honey for the best and most natural taste.

Bread Pan Ingredients:

250ml water
20g low fat olive spread
1 tbsp runny honey
1 ½ tsp salt
1 tbsp skimmed milk powder
45g cracked wheat
440g strong white bread flour
1 ½ tsp fast action dried yeast

Extra Ingredients:

45g pumpkin seeds

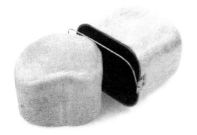

Mozzarella & Basil Bread
750g Loaf

Bread Pan Ingredients:

315ml water
20g low fat olive spread
1 ½ tsp salt
1 ½ tsp 'half spoon' Silver Spoon sugar
1 tbsp skimmed milk powder
600g strong white bread flour
1 ½ tsp fast action dried yeast

Extra Ingredients:

75g finely chopped low fat mozzarella cheese
1 tbsp dried basil

Method:

• Evenly add each bread pan ingredient to the bread maker.
• Add one at a time in the order listed.
• Add the extra ingredients to the dispenser.
• Select the basic program on the bread machine for a 750g loaf.
• Select the crust colour and press start.
• When the baking cycle has finished lift the bread pan out of the machine with oven gloves.
• Turn the baked bread out onto a wire rack to cool.

Using low fat mozzarella helps reduce the calories in this cheesy loaf.

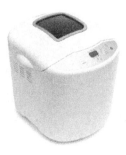

Italian Bread
750g Loaf

Method:

• Evenly add all the ingredients to the bread maker.
• Add each ingredient one at a time in the order listed.
• Select the basic program on the bread machine for a 750g loaf.
• Select the crust colour and press start.
• When the baking cycle has finished lift the bread pan out of the machine with oven gloves.
• Turn the baked bread out onto a wire rack to cool.

Ingredients:

315ml water
2 tbsp olive oil
1 garlic clove, crushed
1 tbsp dried basil
1 tbsp freshly chopped flat leaf parsley
1 ½ tsp salt
1 ½ tsp 'half spoon' Silver Spoon sugar
1 tbsp skimmed milk powder
600g strong white bread flour
1 ½ tsp fast action dried yeast

With its lower saturated fats, baking with olive oil is a good healthier option.

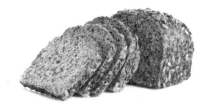

45

Fat Free Yoghurt & Chilli Bread
750g Loaf

Ingredients:

215ml water
125ml fat free Greek yoghurt
1 tbsp cayenne pepper
1 ½ tsp salt
1 ½ tsp 'half spoon' Silver Spoon sugar
1 tbsp skimmed milk powder
440g strong white bread flour
1 ½ tsp fast action dried yeast

Method:

• Evenly add all the ingredients to the bread maker.
• Add each ingredient one at a time in the order listed.
• Select the basic program on the bread machine for a 750g loaf.
• Select the crust colour and press start.
• When the baking cycle has finished lift the bread pan out of the machine with oven gloves.
• Turn the baked bread out onto a wire rack to cool.

Fat free Greek yoghurt is a good 'skinny' alternative to crème fraiche and sour cream in baking.

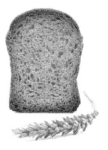

46

Garlic & Oregano Bread
750g Loaf

Method:

- Evenly add all the ingredients to the bread maker.
- Add each ingredient one at a time in the order listed.
- Select the basic program on the bread machine for a 750g loaf.
- Select the crust colour and press start.
- When the baking cycle has finished lift the bread pan out of the machine with oven gloves.
- Turn the baked bread out onto a wire rack to cool.

Basil makes a good alternative to oregano if you prefer.

Ingredients:

315ml water
20g low fat olive spread
2 garlic cloves, crushed
1 tbsp dried oregano
1 ½ tsp salt
1 ½ tsp 'half spoon' Silver Spoon sugar
1 tbsp skimmed milk powder
600g strong white bread flour
1 ½ tsp fast action dried yeast

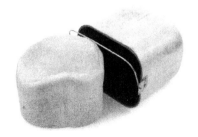

Sundried Tomato Bread
750g Loaf

Ingredients:

315ml water
15g low fat olive spread
1 ½ tbsp sundried tomato puree
1 ½ tsp salt
1 ½ tsp 'half spoon' Silver Spoon sugar
2 tbsp skimmed milk powder
600g strong white bread flour
1 ½ tsp fast action dried yeast

Method:

• Evenly add all the ingredients to the bread maker.
• Add each ingredient one at a time in the order listed.
• Select the basic program on the bread machine for a 750g loaf.
• Select the crust colour and press start.
• When the baking cycle has finished lift the bread pan out of the machine with oven gloves.
• Turn the baked bread out onto a wire rack to cool.

You could also add some chopped sundried tomatoes to the extra ingredients dispenser if you like.

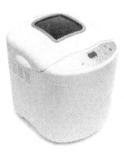

Four Herb Bread
750g Loaf

Method:

• Evenly add all the ingredients to the bread maker.
• Add each ingredient one at a time in the order listed.
• Select the basic program on the bread machine for a 750g loaf.
• Select the crust colour and press start.
• When the baking cycle has finished lift the bread pan out of the machine with oven gloves.
• Turn the baked bread out onto a wire rack to cool.

Feel free to alter the balance of herbs to suit your own taste.

Ingredients:

315ml water
25g low fat olive spread
1 tsp each dried basil, oregano, thyme & rosemary
1 ½ tsp salt
1 ½ tsp 'half spoon' Silver Spoon sugar
1 tbsp skimmed milk powder
600g strong white bread flour
1 ½ tsp fast action dried yeast

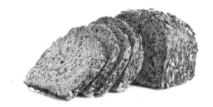

Mediterranean Rosemary Bread
750g Loaf

Ingredients:

265ml water
2 tbsp olive oil
2 tsp dried rosemary
1 ½ tsp salt
1 ½ tsp 'half spoon'
Silver Spoon sugar
1 tbsp skimmed milk
powder
600g strong white bread
flour
1 ½ tsp fast action dried
yeast

Method:

• Evenly add all the ingredients to the bread maker.
• Add each ingredient one at a time in the order listed.
• Select the basic program on the bread machine for a 750g loaf.
• Select the crust colour and press start.
• When the baking cycle has finished lift the bread pan out of the machine with oven gloves.
• Turn the baked bread out onto a wire rack to cool.

The loaf is lovely sprinkled with coarse sea salt after baking.

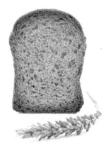

Olive Bread
750g Loaf

Method:

- Evenly add each bread pan ingredient to the bread maker.
- Add one at a time in the order listed.
- Add the chopped olives to the dispenser.
- Select the basic program on the bread machine for a 750g loaf.
- Select the crust colour and press start.
- When the baking cycle has finished lift the bread pan out of the machine with oven gloves.
- Turn the baked bread out onto a wire rack to cool.

Deriving from Greece, kalamata olives have a smooth meaty texture, which works really well in bread.

Bread Pan Ingredients:

315ml water
20g low fat olive spread
1 ½ tsp salt
1 ½ tsp 'half spoon' Silver Spoon sugar
2 tbsp skimmed milk powder
600g strong white bread flour
1 ½ tsp fast action dried yeast

Extra Ingredients:

3 tbsp chopped kalamata olives

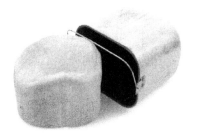

51

Thyme & Lemon Bread
750g Loaf

Ingredients:

315ml water
20g low fat olive spread
1 tbsp dried thyme
1 tbsp lemon zest
1 ½ tsp salt
1 ½ tsp 'half spoon' Silver Spoon sugar
1 tbsp skimmed milk powder
600g strong white bread flour
1 ½ tsp fast action dried yeast

Method:

• Evenly add all the ingredients to the bread maker.
• Add each ingredient one at a time in the order listed.
• Select the basic program on the bread machine for a 750g loaf.
• Select the crust colour and press start.
• When the baking cycle has finished lift the bread pan out of the machine with oven gloves.
• Turn the baked bread out onto a wire rack to cool.

Turn your loaf on the side and you'll find it easier to cut into even slices.

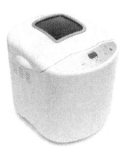

Red Onion Bread
750g Loaf

Method:

- Evenly add all the ingredients to the bread maker.
- Add each ingredient one at a time in the order listed.
- Select the basic program on the bread machine for a 750g loaf.
- Select the crust colour and press start.
- When the baking cycle has finished lift the bread pan out of the machine with oven gloves.
- Turn the baked bread out onto a wire rack to cool.

It's best to quickly sauté the onions in a little low cal cooking oil spray for a few minutes before adding to the bread machine.

Ingredients:

315ml water
20g low fat olive spread
½ red onion, finely chopped
1 ½ tsp salt
1 ½ tsp 'half spoon' Silver Spoon sugar
1 tbsp skimmed milk powder
600g strong white bread flour
1 ½ tsp fast action dried yeast

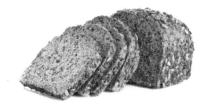

Indian Spiced Bread
750g Loaf

Ingredients:

315ml water
20g low fat olive spread
2 tsp ground turmeric
1 tsp each ground coriander & cumin
1 ½ tsp salt
1 ½ tsp 'half spoon' Silver Spoon sugar
1 tbsp skimmed milk powder
600g strong white bread flour
1 ½ tsp fast action dried yeast

Method:

• Evenly add all the ingredients to the bread maker.
• Add each ingredient one at a time in the order listed.
• Select the basic program on the bread machine for a 750g loaf.
• Select the crust colour and press start.
• When the baking cycle has finished lift the bread pan out of the machine with oven gloves.
• Turn the baked bread out onto a wire rack to cool.

The turmeric in this recipe gives the bread a lovely yellow colour.

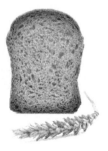

Chorizo & Mozzarella Bread
750g Loaf

Method:

• Evenly add all the ingredients to the bread maker.
• Add each ingredient one at a time in the order listed.
• Select the basic program on the bread machine for a 750g loaf.
• Select the crust colour and press start.
• When the baking cycle has finished lift the bread pan out of the machine with oven gloves.
• Turn the baked bread out onto a wire rack to cool.

Using low fat mozzarella is a 'skinnier' option than the full fat version.

Ingredients:

315ml water
20g low fat olive spread
2 tsp dried basil
70g chopped chorizo
45g shredded low fat mozzarella cheese
1 ½ tsp salt
1 ½ tsp 'half spoon' Silver Spoon sugar
1 tbsp skimmed milk powder
600g strong white bread flour
1 ½ tsp fast action dried yeast

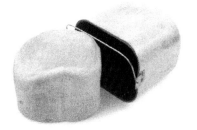

Double Seed Lemon Bread
750g Loaf

Ingredients:

315ml water
20g low fat olive spread
1 tbsp lemon zest
1 tbsp poppy seeds
1 tbsp sesame seeds
1 ½ tsp salt
1 ½ tsp 'half spoon'
Silver Spoon sugar
1 tbsp skimmed milk
powder
600g strong white bread
flour
1 ½ tsp fast action dried
yeast

Method:

• Evenly add all the ingredients to the bread maker.
• Add each ingredient one at a time in the order listed.
• Select the basic program on the bread machine for a 750g loaf.
• Select the crust colour and press start.
• When the baking cycle has finished lift the bread pan out of the machine with oven gloves.
• Turn the baked bread out onto a wire rack to cool.

Poppy seeds have very high nutritional qualities and are generally less allergenic than most other seeds and nuts.

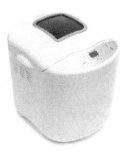

Bacon & Mustard Bread
750g Loaf

Method:

• Evenly add all the ingredients to the bread maker.
• Add each ingredient one at a time in the order listed.
• Select the basic program on the bread machine for a 750g loaf.
• Select the crust colour and press start.
• When the baking cycle has finished lift the bread pan out of the machine with oven gloves.
• Turn the baked bread out onto a wire rack to cool.

Trimming the bacon of any fat will make for less calories.

Ingredients:

315ml water
20g low fat olive spread
3 slices lean, cooked back bacon, finely chopped
2 tsp English mustard powder
1 ½ tsp salt
1 ½ tsp 'half spoon' Silver Spoon sugar
1 tbsp skimmed milk powder
600g strong white bread flour
1 ½ tsp fast action dried yeast

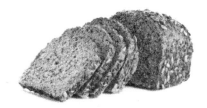

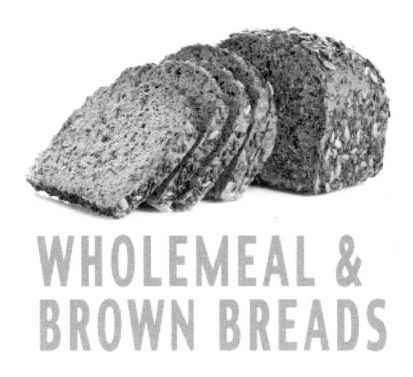

WHOLEMEAL & BROWN BREADS

Granary Grain Bread
750g Loaf

Ingredients:

370ml water
25g low fat olive spread
120g bread grain mix
1 ½ tsp salt
2 ½ tsp 'half spoon'
Silver Spoon sugar
2 tbsp skimmed milk
powder
540g strong wholemeal
bread flour
1 ½ tsp fast action dried
yeast

Method:

• Evenly add all the ingredients to the bread maker.
• Add each ingredient one at a time in the order listed.
• Select the basic wheat program on the bread machine for a 750g loaf.
• Select the crust colour and press start.
• When the baking cycle has finished lift the bread pan out of the machine with oven gloves.
• Turn the baked bread out onto a wire rack to cool.

Bread grain mix is readily available at most health food shops.

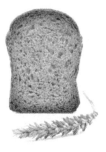

Raisin & Pecan Bread
750g Loaf

Method:

• Evenly add each bread pan ingredient to the bread maker.
• Add one at a time in the order listed.
• Add the extra ingredients to the dispenser.
• Select the basic wheat program on the bread machine for a 750g loaf.
• Select the crust colour and press start.
• When the baking cycle has finished lift the bread pan out of the machine with oven gloves.
• Turn the baked bread out onto a wire rack to cool.

You could use sultanas in this recipe if you prefer.

Bread Pan Ingredients:

320ml water
25g low fat olive spread
1 ½ tsp salt
2 ½ tsp 'half spoon' Silver Spoon sugar
2 tbsp skimmed milk powder
540g strong wholemeal bread flour
1 ½ tsp fast action dried yeast

Extra Ingredients:

75g raisins, chopped
75g pecan nuts, chopped

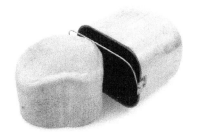

Caraway Rye Bread
750g Loaf

Ingredients:

300ml water
20g low fat olive spread
1 ½ tsp salt
2 ½ tsp 'half spoon'
Silver Spoon sugar
1 tbsp caraway seeds
1 tbsp skimmed milk
powder
400g strong wholemeal
bread flour
160g rye flour
1 ½ tsp fast action dried
yeast

Method:

• Evenly add all the ingredients to the bread maker.
• Add each ingredient one at a time in the order listed.
• Select the basic wheat program on the bread machine for a 750g loaf.
• Select the crust colour and press start.
• When the baking cycle has finished lift the bread pan out of the machine with oven gloves.
• Turn the baked bread out onto a wire rack to cool.

Rye bread is often made using molasses. This skinnier version leaves it out but tastes just as good.

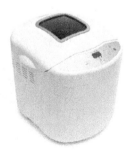

Granola Loaf
750g Loaf

Method:

- Evenly add each bread pan ingredient to the bread maker.
- Add one at a time in the order listed.
- Add the granola to the dispenser.
- Select the basic wheat program on the bread machine for a 750g loaf.
- Select the crust colour and press start.
- When the baking cycle has finished lift the bread pan out of the machine with oven gloves.
- Turn the baked bread out onto a wire rack to cool.

Use unsweetened granola for this recipe.

Bread Pan Ingredients:

320ml water
20g low fat olive spread
1 ½ tsp salt
2 ½ tsp 'half spoon' Silver Spoon sugar
1 tbsp skimmed milk powder
220g strong wholemeal bread flour
320g strong white bread flour
1 ½ tsp fast action dried yeast

Extra Ingredients:

120g granola

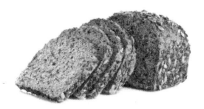

63

Sweet Fennel Bread
750g Loaf

Ingredients:

300ml water
20g low fat olive spread
1 tbsp fennel seeds
3 tsp 'half spoon' Silver Spoon sugar
1 ½ tsp salt
120g rye flour
120g strong wholemeal bread flour
200g strong plain white flour
1 ½ tsp fast action dried yeast

Method:

• Evenly add all the ingredients to the bread maker.
• Add each ingredient one at a time in the order listed.
• Select the basic wheat program on the bread machine for a 750g loaf.
• Select the crust colour and press start.
• When the baking cycle has finished lift the bread pan out of the machine with oven gloves.
• Turn the baked bread out onto a wire rack to cool.

As well as tasting great, fennel is prized in ancient culture for its medicinal properties.

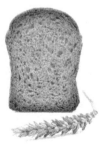

64

Orange & Poppy Seed Bread
750g Loaf

Method:

• Evenly add all the ingredients to the bread maker.
• Add each ingredient one at a time in the order listed.
• Select the basic wheat program on the bread machine for a 750g loaf.
• Select the crust colour and press start.
• When the baking cycle has finished lift the bread pan out of the machine with oven gloves.
• Turn the baked bread out onto a wire rack to cool.

Let the bread cool as much as possible before cutting so that it can be sliced thinly and evenly.

Ingredients:

320ml water
25g low fat olive spread
1 ½ tsp salt
2 ½ tsp 'half spoon' Silver Spoon sugar
1 ½ tsp grated orange zest
1 ½ tsp poppy seeds
2 tbsp skimmed milk powder
540g strong wholemeal bread flour
1 ½ tsp fast action dried yeast

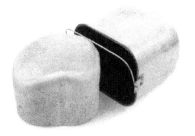

Rye & Cocoa Bread
750g Loaf

Ingredients:

320ml water
25g low fat olive spread
2 tbsp skimmed milk powder
2 tbsp unsweetened cocoa powder
2 ½ tsp 'half spoon' Silver Spoon sugar
1 ½ tsp salt
120g rye flour
420g strong wholemeal bread flour
1 ½ tsp fast action dried yeast

Method:

• Evenly add all the ingredients to the bread maker.
• Add each ingredient one at a time in the order listed.
• Select the basic wheat program on the bread machine for a 750g loaf.
• Select the crust colour and press start.
• When the baking cycle has finished lift the bread pan out of the machine with oven gloves.
• Turn the baked bread out onto a wire rack to cool.

The rye flour will make this loaf fairly dense, so make sure you slice it really thinly.

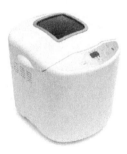

Honey & Pumpkin Seed Loaf
750g Loaf

Method:

• Evenly add each bread pan ingredient to the bread maker.
• Add one at a time in the order listed.
• Add the pumpkin seeds to the dispenser.
• Select the basic wheat program on the bread machine for a 750g loaf.
• Select the crust colour and press start.
• When the baking cycle has finished lift the bread pan out of the machine with oven gloves.
• Turn the baked bread out onto a wire rack to cool.

Oatmeal provides additional fibre and texture to the loaf.

Bread Pan Ingredients:

275ml water
25g low fat olive spread
1 ½ tsp salt
1 tbsp runny honey
1 tbsp skimmed milk powder
220g strong white bread flour
160g strong wholemeal bread flour
85g oatmeal
1 ½ tsp fast action dried yeast

Extra Ingredients:

85g pumpkin seeds

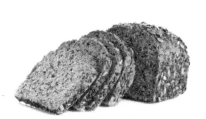

Cinnamon & Carrot Bread
750g Loaf

Ingredients:

300ml water
20g low fat olive spread
3 tbsp grated carrot
1 tbsp ground cinnamon
3 tsp 'half spoon' Silver Spoon sugar
1 ½ tsp salt
1 tbsp skimmed milk powder
240g strong wholemeal bread flour
200g strong white bread flour
1 ½ tsp fast action dried yeast

Method:

• Evenly add all the ingredients to the bread maker.
• Add each ingredient one at a time in the order listed.
• Select the basic wheat program on the bread machine for a 750g loaf.
• Select the crust colour and press start.
• When the baking cycle has finished lift the bread pan out of the machine with oven gloves.
• Turn the baked bread out onto a wire rack to cool.

Carrots & cinnamon make a great combination in this mixed-flour bread.

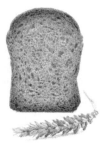

Almond & Syrup Bread
750g Loaf

Method:

• Evenly add all the ingredients to the bread maker.
• Add each ingredient one at a time in the order listed.
• Select the basic wheat program on the bread machine for a 750g loaf.
• Select the crust colour and press start.
• When the baking cycle has finished lift the bread pan out of the machine with oven gloves.
• Turn the baked bread out onto a wire rack to cool.

The almonds give a little crunch to this bread whilst the agave syrup provides natural sweetness.

Ingredients:

320ml water
25g low fat olive spread
75g chopped almonds
1 ½ tsp salt
2 tbsp agave syrup
2 tbsp skimmed milk powder
540g strong wholemeal bread flour
1 ½ tsp fast action dried yeast

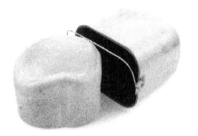

Oaty Bread
750g Loaf

Ingredients:

275ml water
25g low fat olive spread
1 ½ tsp salt
200g strong white bread flour
250g strong wholemeal bread flour
50g rolled oats
1 tbsp agave syrup
2 tsp fast action dried yeast

Method:

• Evenly add all the ingredients to the bread maker.
• Add each ingredient one at a time in the order listed.
• Select the basic wheat program on the bread machine for a 750g loaf.
• Select the crust colour and press start.
• When the baking cycle has finished lift the bread pan out of the machine with oven gloves.
• Turn the baked bread out onto a wire rack to cool.

Rolled oats are a great source of iron, thiamine and dietary fibre.

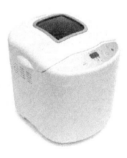

Barley Milk Bread
750g Loaf

Method:

• Evenly add all the ingredients to the bread maker.
• Add each ingredient one at a time in the order listed.
• Select the basic wheat program on the bread machine for a 750g loaf.
• Select the crust colour and press start.
• When the baking cycle has finished lift the bread pan out of the machine with oven gloves.
• Turn the baked bread out onto a wire rack to cool.

Used widely in health foods, barley contains eight essential amino acids.

Ingredients:

275ml water
2 tbsp skimmed milk powder
25g low fat olive spread
2 tsp 'half spoon' Silver Spoon sugar
1 ½ tsp salt
475g strong wholemeal bread flour
50g barley flakes
1 ½ tsp fast action dried yeast

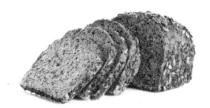

Triple Seed Bread
750g Loaf

Ingredients:

275ml water
2 tbsp skimmed milk powder
2 tbsp sunflower oil
1 ½ tsp salt
2 tsp 'half spoon' Silver Spoon sugar
1 tbsp each pumpkin, sunflower & flax seeds
275g strong wholemeal bread flour
200g strong white bread flour
1 ½ tsp fast action dried yeast

Method:

• Evenly add all the ingredients to the bread maker.
• Add each ingredient one at a time in the order listed.
• Select the basic wheat program on the bread machine for a 750g loaf.
• Select the crust colour and press start.
• When the baking cycle has finished lift the bread pan out of the machine with oven gloves.
• Turn the baked bread out onto a wire rack to cool.

Flax seeds contain high levels of dietary fibre and micronutrients.

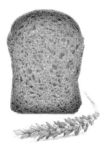

Granary & Stout Loaf
750g Loaf

Method:

• Evenly add all the ingredients to the bread maker.
• Add each ingredient one at a time in the order listed.
• Select the basic wheat program on the bread machine for a 750g loaf.
• Select the crust colour and press start.
• When the baking cycle has finished lift the bread pan out of the machine with oven gloves.
• Turn the baked bread out onto a wire rack to cool.

Granary flour adds a lovely malty taste to this loaf.

Ingredients:

200ml stout
100ml water
2 tbsp vegetable oil
1 ½ tsp salt
3 tsp 'half spoon' Silver Spoon sugar
475g granary flour
200g strong white bread flour
1 ½ tsp fast action dried yeast

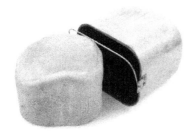

Lemon & Parsley Bread
750g Loaf

Ingredients:

200ml water
1 tsp grated lemon zest
150g fat free Greek yoghurt
1 ½ tsp salt
1 ½ tsp 'half spoon' Silver Spoon sugar
2 tbsp dried parsley
500g strong wholemeal bread flour
1 ½ tsp fast action dried yeast

Method:

• Evenly add all the ingredients to the bread maker.
• Add each ingredient one at a time in the order listed.
• Select the basic wheat program on the bread machine for a 750g loaf.
• Select the crust colour and press start.
• When the baking cycle has finished lift the bread pan out of the machine with oven gloves.
• Turn the baked bread out onto a wire rack to cool.

Fat free yoghurt is a great 'skinny' alternative to sour cream.

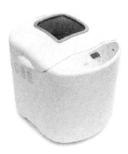

74

Walnut Bread
750g Loaf

Method:

- Evenly add each bread pan ingredient to the bread maker.
- Add one at a time in the order listed.
- Add the extra ingredients to the dispenser.
- Select the basic wheat program on the bread machine for a 750g loaf.
- Select the crust colour and press start.
- When the baking cycle has finished lift the bread pan out of the machine with oven gloves.
- Turn the baked bread out onto a wire rack to cool.

Chop the walnuts quite finely to spread them through the loaf.

Bread Pan Ingredients:

220ml water
100ml skimmed milk
25g low fat olive spread
1 ½ tsp salt
2 ½ tsp 'half spoon' Silver Spoon sugar
2 tbsp skimmed milk powder
540g strong wholemeal bread flour
1 ½ tsp fast action dried yeast

Extra Ingredients:

50g chopped walnuts

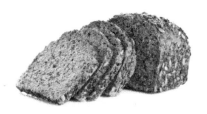

Granary Linseed Bread
750g Loaf

Ingredients:

300ml water
30g low fat olive spread
2 tbsp skimmed milk powder
1 ½ tsp 'half spoon' Silver Spoon sugar
1 ½ tsp salt
475g granary flour
3 tbsp linseeds
1 ½ tsp fast action dried yeast

Method:

• Evenly add all the ingredients to the bread maker.
• Add each ingredient one at a time in the order listed.
• Select the basic wheat program on the bread machine for a 750g loaf.
• Select the crust colour and press start.
• When the baking cycle has finished lift the bread pan out of the machine with oven gloves.
• Turn the baked bread out onto a wire rack to cool.

This is a good loaf to set the timer for as it doesn't use fresh ingredients.

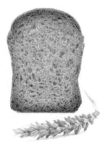

German Seed Bread
750g Loaf

Method:

- Evenly add all the ingredients to the bread maker.
- Add each ingredient one at a time in the order listed.
- Select the basic wheat program on the bread machine for a 750g loaf.
- Select the crust colour and press start.
- When the baking cycle has finished lift the bread pan out of the machine with oven gloves.
- Turn the baked bread out onto a wire rack to cool.

This seeded loaf will have quite a dense texture so be sure to slice it thinly.

Ingredients:

300ml water
2 tbsp olive oil
1 ½ tsp salt
1 ½ tsp 'half spoon'
Silver Spoon sugar
50g pumpkin seeds
2 tbsp skimmed milk
powder
475g strong wholemeal
bread flour
1 ½ tsp fast action dried
yeast

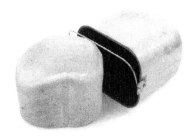

Dried Chilli Bread
750g Loaf

Ingredients:

320ml water
30g low fat olive spread
1 ½ tsp salt
1 tbsp crushed chilli flakes
2 tsp 'half spoon' Silver Spoon sugar
2 tbsp skimmed milk powder
540g strong wholemeal bread flour
1 ½ tsp fast action dried yeast

Method:

• Evenly add all the ingredients to the bread maker.
• Add each ingredient one at a time in the order listed.
• Select the basic wheat program on the bread machine for a 750g loaf.
• Select the crust colour and press start.
• When the baking cycle has finished lift the bread pan out of the machine with oven gloves.
• Turn the baked bread out onto a wire rack to cool.

You could also use whole dried chillies in this recipe if you chop them finely enough.

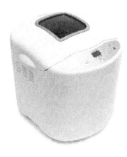

Malthouse Bread
750g Loaf

Method:

• Evenly add all the ingredients to the bread maker.
• Add each ingredient one at a time in the order listed.
• Select the basic wheat program on the bread machine for a 750g loaf.
• Select the crust colour and press start.
• When the baking cycle has finished lift the bread pan out of the machine with oven gloves.
• Turn the baked bread out onto a wire rack to cool.

Malthouse flour is a nutty, slightly sweet tasting flour.

Ingredients:

300ml water
25g low fat olive spread
1 ½ tsp salt
2 tsp 'half spoon' Silver Spoon sugar
500g malthouse bread flour
1 ½ tsp fast action dried yeast

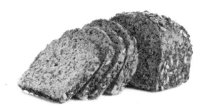

Barleycorn Flour Loaf
750g Loaf

Ingredients:

300ml water
1 tbsp olive oil
1 ½ tsp salt
2 tsp 'half spoon' Silver Spoon sugar
350g barleycorn bread
150g strong white bread flour
1 ½ tsp fast action dried yeast

Method:

• Evenly add all the ingredients to the bread maker.
• Add each ingredient one at a time in the order listed.
• Select the basic wheat program on the bread machine for a 750g loaf.
• Select the crust colour and press start.
• When the baking cycle has finished lift the bread pan out of the machine with oven gloves.
• Turn the baked bread out onto a wire rack to cool.

The mix of barleycorn and white flour should give this loaf a lovely soft texture.

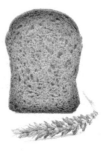

Russian Bread
750g Loaf

Method:

- Evenly add all the ingredients to the bread maker.
- Add each ingredient one at a time in the order listed.
- Select the basic wheat program on the bread machine for a 750g loaf.
- Select the crust colour and press start.
- When the baking cycle has finished lift the bread pan out of the machine with oven gloves.
- Turn the baked bread out onto a wire rack to cool.

This bread should be dark in colour. Slice very thinly and serve with cheese & pickled onions.

Ingredients:

325ml water
20g low fat olive spread
1 ½ tsp salt
2 tsp 'half spoon' Siver Spoon sugar
1 tbsp cocoa powder
1 tbsp instant coffee granules
250g strong wholemeal flour
250g strong white bread flour
1 ½ tsp fast action dried yeast

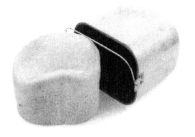

Buckwheat Loaf
750g Loaf

Ingredients:

325ml water
25g low fat olive spread
1 ½ tsp salt
2 tsp 'half spoon' Silver
Spoon sugar
75g buckwheat flour
225g strong wholemeal
flour
200g strong white bread
flour
1 ½ tsp fast action dried
yeast

Method:

• Evenly add all the ingredients to the bread maker.
• Add each ingredient one at a time in the order listed.
• Select the basic wheat program on the bread machine for a 750g loaf.
• Select the crust colour and press start.
• When the baking cycle has finished lift the bread pan out of the machine with oven gloves.
• Turn the baked bread out onto a wire rack to cool.

Buckwheat flour can struggle to rise, so this recipe uses both wholemeal and strong white flour to help the process.

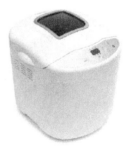

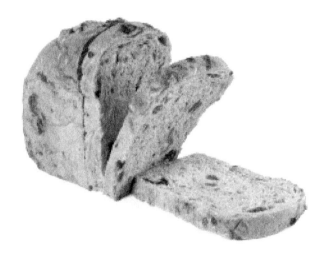

SWEET BREADS

Your bread machine will need a 'sweet' program to bake these breads. These loaves are skinnier versions of popular recipes, but they should still be eaten in moderation if you are counting your calories.

Banana Bread
750g Loaf

Ingredients:

125ml water
30g low fat olive spread
2 bananas, mashed
1 free range egg
1 ½ tsp salt
4 ½ tsp 'half spoon'
Silver Spoon sugar
2 tbsp skimmed milk
powder
520g strong white bread
flour
1 ½ tsp fast action dried
yeast

Method:

• Evenly add all the ingredients to the bread maker.
• Add each ingredient one at a time in the order listed.
• Select the sweet program on the bread machine for a 750g loaf.
• Select the crust colour and press start.
• When the baking cycle has finished lift the bread pan out of the machine with oven gloves.
• Turn the baked bread out onto a wire rack to cool.

Use ripe bananas for this recipe to get the best taste.

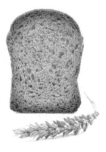

Festive Apple Bread
750g Loaf

Method:

- Evenly add each bread pan ingredient to the bread maker.
- Add one at a time in the order listed.
- Add the apple pieces to the dispenser.
- Select the sweet program on the bread machine for a 750g loaf.
- Select the crust colour and press start.
- When the baking cycle has finished lift the bread pan out of the machine with oven gloves.
- Turn the baked bread out onto a wire rack to cool.

The combination of cinnamon, nutmeg & cloves create an unmistakably festive aroma.

Bread Pan Ingredients:

250ml water
25g low fat olive spread
1 tsp each ground cinnamon & nutmeg
½ tsp ground cloves
1 ½ tsp salt
3 tsp 'half spoon' Silver Spoon sugar
1 tbsp skimmed milk powder
480g strong white bread flour
1 ½ tsp fast action dried yeast

Extra Ingredients:

100g dried apple pieces, finely chopped

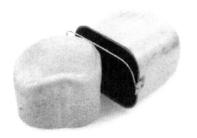

Pineapple & Coconut Bread
750g Loaf

Bread Pan Ingredients:

200ml water
25g low fat olive spread
150g pineapple flesh, finely chopped
1 ½ tsp salt
1 tbsp 'half spoon' Silver Spoon sugar
1 tbsp skimmed milk powder
480g strong white bread flour
2 tsp fast action dried yeast

Extra Ingredients:

120g desiccated coconut

Method:

• Evenly add each bread pan ingredient to the bread maker.
• Add one at a time in the order listed.
• Add the coconut to the dispenser.
• Select the sweet program on the bread machine for a 750g loaf.
• Select the crust colour and press start.
• When the baking cycle has finished lift the bread pan out of the machine with oven gloves.
• Turn the baked bread out onto a wire rack to cool.

You could use drained, tinned pineapple for this recipe too.

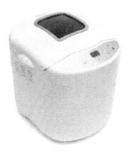

Dried Cherry Loaf
750g Loaf

Method:

- Evenly add each bread pan ingredient to the bread maker.
- Add one at a time in the order listed.
- Add the cherries to the dispenser.
- Select the sweet program on the bread machine for a 750g loaf.
- Select the crust colour and press start.
- When the baking cycle has finished lift the bread pan out of the machine with oven gloves.
- Turn the baked bread out onto a wire rack to cool.

All fresh home baked bread should ideally be eaten within 2-3 days, but can be frozen and stored.

Bread Pan Ingredients:

250ml water
25g low fat olive spread
1 ½ tsp salt
3 tsp 'half spoon' Silver Spoon sugar
480g strong white bread flour
2 tsp fast action dried yeast

Extra Ingredients:

150g dried cherries, chopped

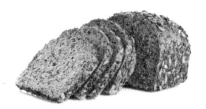

Mixed Fruit & Double Spice Loaf
750g Loaf

Bread Pan Ingredients:

250ml water
20g low fat olive spread
2 tsp nutmeg
1 tsp ground cloves
1 ½ tsp salt
3 tsp half spoon' Silver Spoon sugar
1 tbsp skimmed milk powder
480g strong white bread flour
1 ½ tsp fast action dried yeast

Extra Ingredients:

100g dried mixed fruit, chopped

Method:

• Evenly add each bread pan ingredient to the bread maker.
• Add one at a time in the order listed.
• Add the mixed fruit to the dispenser.
• Select the sweet program on the bread machine for a 750g loaf.
• Select the crust colour and press start.
• When the baking cycle has finished lift the bread pan out of the machine with oven gloves.
• Turn the baked bread out onto a wire rack to cool.

Make sure you use tepid room-temperature water in your bread recipes.

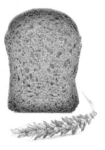

Macadamia & Syrup Loaf
750g Loaf

Method:

• Evenly add each bread pan ingredient to the bread maker.
• Add one at a time in the order listed.
• Add the nuts to the dispenser.
• Select the sweet program on the bread machine for a 750g loaf.
• Select the crust colour and press start.
• When the baking cycle has finished lift the bread pan out of the machine with oven gloves.
• Turn the baked bread out onto a wire rack to cool.

Bread Pan Ingredients:

220ml water
20g low fat olive spread
1 ½ tsp salt
2 tbsp agave syrup
480g strong white bread flour
1 ½ tsp fast action dried yeast

Extra Ingredients:

100g chopped macadamia nuts

Make sure the yeast you use is 'in date' for all your baking. Old yeast will give inferior results.

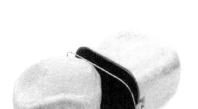

Ginger Raisin Bread
750g Loaf

Bread Pan Ingredients:

250ml water
20g low fat olive spread
1 ½ tsp salt
2 tbsp agave syrup
1 tbsp ground ginger
480g strong white bread flour
2 tsp fast action dried yeast

Extra Ingredients:

120g chopped raisins or sultanas

Method:

• Evenly add each bread pan ingredient to the bread maker.
• Add one at a time in the order listed.
• Add the raisins to the dispenser.
• Select the sweet program on the bread machine for a 750g loaf.
• Select the crust colour and press start.
• When the baking cycle has finished lift the bread pan out of the machine with oven gloves.
• Turn the baked bread out onto a wire rack to cool.

You could substitute good quality honey for agave syrup in this recipe.

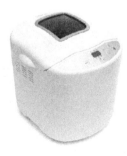

Apricot & Cinnamon Bread
750g Loaf

Method:

- Evenly add each bread pan ingredient to the bread maker.
- Add one at a time in the order listed.
- Add the apricots to the dispenser.
- Select the sweet program on the bread machine for a 750g loaf.
- Select the crust colour and press start.
- When the baking cycle has finished lift the bread pan out of the machine with oven gloves.
- Turn the baked bread out onto a wire rack to cool.

Apricots and cinnamon are a lovely combination. This bread is delicious served with reduced fat cheese.

Bread Pan Ingredients:

250ml water
20g low fat olive spread
1 tbsp cinnamon
1 ½ tsp salt
3 tsp 'half spoon' Silver Spoon sugar
1 tbsp skimmed milk powder
480g strong white bread flour
2 tsp dried yeast

Extra Ingredients:

180g dried apricots, chopped

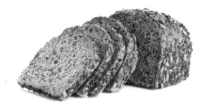

Peanut Butter Bread
750g Loaf

Ingredients:

250ml water
3 tbsp low fat peanut butter
1 ½ tsp salt
2 tsp 'half spoon' Silver Spoon sugar
2 tbsp skimmed milk powder
480g strong white bread flour
2 tsp fast action dried yeast

Method:

• Evenly add all the ingredients to the bread maker.
• Add each ingredient one at a time in the order listed.
• Select the sweet program on the bread machine for a 750g loaf.
• Select the crust colour and press start.
• When the baking cycle has finished lift the bread pan out of the machine with oven gloves.
• Turn the baked bread out onto a wire rack to cool.

Use low fat smooth peanut butter rather than crunchy peanut butter for this recipe.

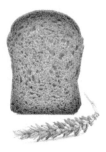

Honey Porridge Loaf
750g Loaf

Method:

• Evenly add all the ingredients to the bread maker.
• Add each ingredient one at a time in the order listed.
• Select the sweet program on the bread machine for a 750g loaf.
• Select the crust colour and press start.
• When the baking cycle has finished lift the bread pan out of the machine with oven gloves.
• Turn the baked bread out onto a wire rack to cool.

Make sure you use a kitchen measuring spoon to get accurate measurements for your baking.

Ingredients:

270ml water
20g low fat olive spread
120g porridge oats
1 ½ tsp salt
1 tbsp runny honey
2 tbsp skimmed milk powder
480g strong white bread flour
2 tsp fast action dried yeast

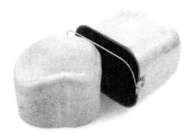

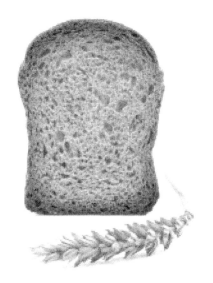

GLUTEN FREE BREADS

This small selection of breads are gluten free. A notable percentage of people have a gluten intolerance which makes eating ordinary bread uncomfortable. Gluten free baking can be a little more temperamental, but practice makes perfect!

Rice Bread
1.25kg Loaf

Ingredients:

500ml water
1 ½ tsp salt
3 free range eggs
80ml olive oil
1 tsp white wine vinegar
480g rice flour
150g cornflour
1 tbsp xanthan gum
1 tbsp 'half spoon' Silver Spoon sugar
2 tsp fast action dried yeast

Method:

• Evenly add all the ingredients to the bread maker.
• Add each ingredient one at a time in the order listed.
• Select the gluten free program on the bread machine for a 1.25kg loaf.
• Select the crust colour and press start.
• When the baking cycle has finished lift the bread pan out of the machine with oven gloves.
• Turn the baked bread out onto a wire rack to cool.

It is normal for gluten free loaves to be denser than your usual loaf.

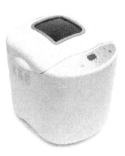

Cinnamon Mixed Fruit Loaf
1.25kg Loaf

Method:

• Evenly add each bread pan ingredient to the bread maker.
• Add one at a time in the order listed.
• Add the mixed fruit to the dispenser.
• Select the gluten free program on the bread machine for a 1.25kg loaf.
• Select the crust colour and press start.
• When the baking cycle has finished lift the bread pan out of the machine with oven gloves.
• Turn the baked bread out onto a wire rack to cool.

Xanthan gum helps with the texture of the loaf by replacing some of the elasticity of the missing gluten.

Bread Pan Ingredients:

470ml water
1 ½ tsp salt
3 free range eggs
80ml olive oil
1 tsp white wine vinegar
480g rice flour
150g cornflour
1 tbsp xanthan gum
1 tbsp 'half spoon' Silver Spoon sugar
1 tbsp runny honey
2 tsp ground cinnamon
2 tsp fast action dried yeast

Extra Ingredients:

150g dried mixed fruit, chopped

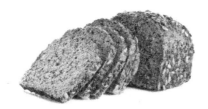

Mixed Seed Bread
1kg Loaf

Bread Pan Ingredients:

500ml water
1 ½ tsp salt
3 free range eggs
80ml olive oil
1 tsp white wine vinegar
480g rice flour
150g cornflour
1 tbsp xanthan gum
1 tbsp 'half spoon' Silver Spoon sugar

Extra Ingredients:

100g mixed seeds

Method:

• Evenly add each bread pan ingredient to the bread maker.
• Add one at a time in the order listed.
• Add the seeds to the dispenser.
• Select the gluten free program on the bread machine for a 1kg loaf.
• Select the crust colour and press start.
• When the baking cycle has finished lift the bread pan out of the machine with oven gloves.
• Turn the baked bread out onto a wire rack to cool.

Packets of mixed seeds (pumpkin, sunflower seeds etc) are available from most supermarkets & health food stores.

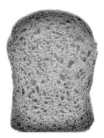

Besan Bread
1kg Loaf

Method:

- Evenly add all the ingredients to the bread maker.
- Add each ingredient one at a time in the order listed.
- Select the gluten free program on the bread machine for a 1kg loaf.
- Select the crust colour and press start.
- When the baking cycle has finished lift the bread pan out of the machine with oven gloves.
- Turn the baked bread out onto a wire rack to cool.

Ingredients:

470ml water
1 ½ tsp salt
3 free range eggs
80ml olive oil
1 tsp white wine vinegar
400g rice flour
80g chickpea flour
150g cornflour
1 tbsp xanthan gum
1 tbsp 'half spoon' Silver Spoon sugar
2 tsp fast action dried yeast

Besan and garbanzo are both alternative names for chickpeas. This loaf uses a blend of both chickpea and rice flours.

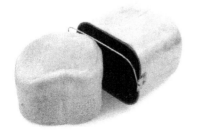

CONVERSION CHART: DRY INGREDIENTS

Metric	Imperial
7g	¼ oz
15g	½ oz
20g	¾ oz
25g	1 oz
40g	1½oz
50g	2oz
60g	2½oz
75g	3oz
100g	3½oz
125g	4oz
140g	4½oz
150g	5oz
165g	5½oz
175g	6oz
200g	7oz
225g	8oz
250g	9oz
275g	10oz
300g	11oz
350g	12oz
375g	13oz
400g	14oz

Metric	Imperial
425g	15oz
450g	1lb
500g	1lb 2oz
550g	1¼lb
600g	1lb 5oz
650g	1lb 7oz
675g	1½lb
700g	1lb 9oz
750g	1lb 11oz
800g	1¾lb
900g	2lb
1kg	2¼lb
1.1kg	2½lb
1.25kg	2¾lb
1.35kg	3lb
1.5kg	3lb 6oz
1.8kg	4lb
2kg	4½lb
2.25kg	5lb
2.5kg	5½lb
2.75kg	6lb

CONVERSION CHART: LIQUID MEASURES

Metric	Imperial	US
25ml	1fl oz	
60ml	2fl oz	¼ cup
75ml	2½ fl oz	
100ml	3½fl oz	
120ml	4fl oz	½ cup
150ml	5fl oz	
175ml	6fl oz	
200ml	7fl oz	
250ml	8½ fl oz	1 cup
300ml	10½ fl oz	
360ml	12½ fl oz	
400ml	14fl oz	
450ml	15½ fl oz	
600ml	1 pint	
750ml	1¼ pint	3 cups
1 litre	1½ pints	4 cups

Other COOKNATION TITLES

You may also be interested in other titles in the CookNation series. In particular, a perfect companion to Skinny Bread Machine is 'The Skinny Soup Maker Recipe Book: Delicious Low Calorie, Healthy and Simple Soup Machine Recipes Under 100, 200 and 300 Calories. Perfect For Any Diet and Weight Loss Plan.'

If you enjoyed 'The Skinny Bread Machine Recipe Book' we'd really appreciate your feedback. Reviews help others decide if this is the right book for them so a moment of your time would be appreciated.

Thank you.

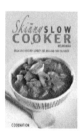

The Skinny Slow Cooker Recipe Book

Delicious Recipes Under 300, 400 And 500 Calories.

Paperback / eBook

More Skinny Slow Cooker Recipes

75 More Delicious Recipes Under 300, 400 & 500 Calories.

Paperback / eBook

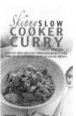

The Skinny Slow Cooker Curry Recipe Book

Low Calorie Curries From Around The World

Paperback / eBook

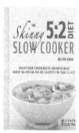

The Skinny Slow Cooker Soup Recipe Book

Simple, Healthy & Delicious Low Calorie Soup Recipes For Your Slow Cooker. All Under 100, 200 & 300 Calories.

Paperback / eBook

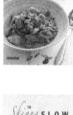

The Skinny Slow Cooker Vegetarian Recipe Book

40 Delicious Recipes Under 200, 300 And 400 Calories.

Paperback / eBook

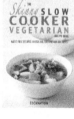

The Skinny 5:2 Slow Cooker Recipe Book

Skinny Slow Cooker Recipe And Menu Ideas Under 100, 200, 300 & 400 Calories For Your 5:2 Diet.

Paperback / eBook

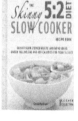

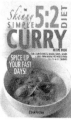

The Skinny 5:2 Curry Recipe Book

Spice Up Your Fast Days With Simple Low Calorie Curries, Snacks, Soups, Salads & Sides Under 200, 300 & 400 Calories

Paperback / eBook

The Skinny Halogen Oven Family Favourites Recipe Book

Healthy, Low Calorie Family Meal-Time Halogen Oven Recipes Under 300, 400 and 500 Calories

Paperback / eBook

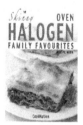

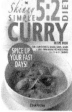

Skinny Halogen Oven Cooking For One

Single Serving, Healthy, Low Calorie Halogen Oven Recipes Under 200, 300 and 400 Calories

Paperback / eBook

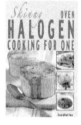

Skinny Winter Warmers Recipe Book

Soups, Stews, Casseroles & One Pot Meals Under 300, 400 & 500 Calories.

Paperback / eBook

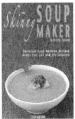

The Skinny Soup Maker Recipe Book

Delicious Low Calorie, Healthy and Simple Soup Recipes Under 100, 200 and 300 Calories. Perfect For Any Diet and Weight Loss Plan.

Paperback / eBook

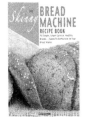

The Skinny Bread Machine Recipe Book

70 Simple, Lower Calorie, Healthy Breads...Baked To Perfection In Your Bread Maker.

Paperback / eBook

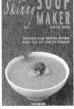

The Skinny Indian Takeaway Recipe Book

Authentic British Indian Restaurant Dishes Under 300, 400 And 500 Calories. The Secret To Low Calorie Indian Takeaway Food At Home

Paperback / eBook

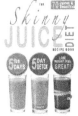

The Skinny Juice Diet Recipe Book

5lbs, 5 Days. The Ultimate Kick-Start Diet and Detox Plan to Lose Weight & Feel Great!

Paperback / eBook

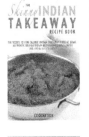

The Skinny 5:2 Diet Recipe Book Collection

All The 5:2 Fast Diet Recipes You'll Ever Need. All Under 100, 200, 300, 400 And 500 Calories

Available only on eBook

eBook

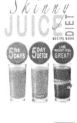

The Skinny 5:2 Fast Diet Meals For One

Single Serving Fast Day Recipes & Snacks Under 100, 200 & 300 Calories

Paperback / eBook

The Skinny 5:2 Fast Diet Vegetarian Meals For One

Single Serving Fast Day Recipes & Snacks Under 100, 200 & 300 Calories

Paperback / eBook

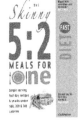

The Skinny 5:2 Fast Diet Family Favourites Recipe Book

Eat With All The Family On Your Diet Fasting Days

Paperback / eBook

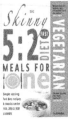

The Skinny 5:2 Fast Diet Family Favorites Recipe Book *U.S.A. EDITION*

Dine With All The Family On Your Diet Fasting Days

Available only on eBook

Paperback / eBook

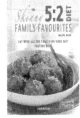

The Skinny 5:2 Diet Chicken Dishes Recipe Book

Delicious Low Calorie Chicken Dishes Under 300, 400 & 500 Calories

Paperback / eBook

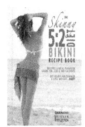

The Skinny 5:2 Bikini Diet Recipe Book

Recipes & Meal Planners Under 100, 200 & 300 Calories. Get Ready For Summer & Lose Weight...FAST!

Paperback / eBook

Available only on eBook

The Paleo Diet For Beginners Slow Cooker Recipe Book

Gluten Free, Everyday Essential Slow Cooker Paleo Recipes For Beginners

eBook

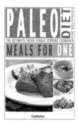

The Paleo Diet For Beginners Meals For One

The Ultimate Paleo Single Serving Cookbook

Paperback / eBook

Available only on eBook

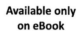

The Paleo Diet For Beginners Holidays

Thanksgiving, Christmas & New Year Paleo Friendly Recipes

eBook

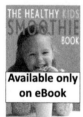

Available only on eBook

The Healthy Kids Smoothie Book

40 Delicious Goodness In A Glass Recipes for Happy Kids.

eBook

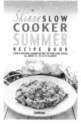

The Skinny Slow Cooker Summer Recipe Book

Fresh & Seasonal Summer Recipes For Your Slow Cooker. All Under 300, 400 And 500 Calories.

Paperback / eBook

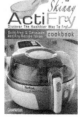
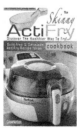

The Skinny ActiFry Cookbook

Guilt-free and Delicious ActiFry Recipe Ideas: Discover The Healthier Way to Fry!

Paperback / eBook

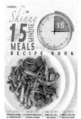

The Skinny 15 Minute Meals Recipe Book

Delicious, Nutritious & Super-Fast Meals in 15 Minutes Or Less. All Under 300, 400 & 500 Calories.

Paperback / eBook

The Skinny Mediterranean Recipe Book

Simple, Healthy & Delicious Low Calorie Mediterranean Diet Dishes. All Under 200, 300 & 400 Calories.

Paperback / eBook

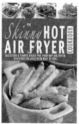

The Skinny Hot Air Fryer Cookbook

Delicious & Simple Meals For Your Hot Air Fryer: Discover The Healthier Way To Fry.

Paperback / eBook

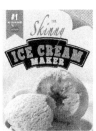

The Skinny Ice Cream Maker

Delicious Lower Fat, Lower Calorie Ice Cream, Frozen Yogurt & Sorbet Recipes For Your Ice Cream Maker

Paperback / eBook

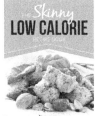

The Skinny Low Calorie Recipe Book

Great Tasting, Simple & Healthy Meals Under 300, 400 & 500 Calories. Perfect For Any Calorie Controlled Diet.

Paperback / eBook

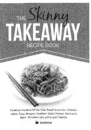

The Skinny Takeaway Recipe Book

Healthier Versions Of Your Fast Food Favourites: Chinese, Indian, Pizza, Burgers, Southern Style Chicken, Mexican & More. All Under 300, 400 & 500 Calories

Paperback / eBook

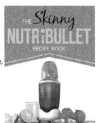

The Skinny Nutribullet Recipe Book

80+ Delicious & Nutritious Healthy Smoothie Recipes. Burn Fat, Lose Weight and Feel Great!

Paperback / eBook

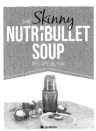

The Skinny Nutribullet Soup Recipe Book

Delicious, Quick & Easy, Single Serving Soups & Pasta Sauces For Your Nutribullet. All Under 100, 200, 300 & 400 Calories.

Paperback / eBook

107

Printed in Great Britain
by Amazon

85909393R10066